The Complete Kombucha Brewing Journal

Neil Stolmaker
Laurie Stolmaker

The Complete Kombucha Brewing Journal
by Neil Stolmaker and Laurie Stolmaker

© Copyright 2016 Neil Stolmaker and Laurie Stolmaker. All Rights Reserved.

Cover, print and interior design by Neil Stolmaker and Laurie Stolmaker.

While every precaution has been taken in the preparation of this book, the publisher and authors assume no responsibility for errors or omissions, or for damages resulting from the use of the information contained herein.

CONTENTS

Getting Started - How to use this journal 4
Kombucha Brewing Diagram 9
Brewing Record Sample 10
Recipe Sample 11
Brewing Records 12
Recipe List 60
Recipes 62
SCOBY Family Tree 86
Inspirations 96
Wellness Notes 100
Purchase Record 104

Getting Started

> **Congratulations on purchasing this journal.**
>
> We have an exciting bonus gift waiting for you. Get our Kombucha Quick Start Guide with our top 10 brewing tips and 6 of our favorite yummy kombucha recipes for free. Go right now and sign up at kombuchajournal.com/readers

Getting Started with the Complete Kombucha Brewing Journal

Brewing Records Pages

Here is where you record the information each time you brew kombucha. You can write down the tea ingredients, the environment in the room, temperature and pH of the brew and other observations and notes about the brewing process, timing and appearance. In the *Steps Table*, you can note down each of the necessary steps that you followed for easy recall. If you are using a heat source on a timer, record that information in the *Steps Table* too.

Brewing Record Pages Fields (see completed sample form on page 10)

Batch #: create a unique number for each batch. It is probably easiest to just start with number one.

BB / CB: Mark whether this batch is a single batch brew, BB or a continuous brew, CB.

Previous Batch #/Page #: If you are continuing this batch from another one, record that Batch # and Page # in this space.

Date Begun: Write down the date that you began to make this batch of kombucha. Sometimes you may make your sweetened tea, but add the SCOBY on a different day.

Date Bottled: When you are ready to bottle your kombucha, record that date here.

Ingredient Table

Ingredient: Write in a complete description of each ingredient. For example, you might write, "English Breakfast black tea blend." Also, you might include the brand or source of the tea.

Amount: Put down how much of each ingredient was used.

Brew Time: Record how long the brew time was for that ingredient. You will want to know how long you brewed each tea ingredient for, although for the sugar, you just stir until dissolved.

Steps Table: This is for your own notes as to how you created your brew.

Added check boxes: Tea, Sugar, Other - The tea, sugar fields are there for you to check off so that you don't forget those vital steps. You can use the other field to write in a different main ingredient, such as honey.

SCOBY Name: Your SCOBY makes kombucha for you, so it is nice to provide it with a name. Before you know it, you will have more than one SCOBY, so you will need a way to keep track of them. Of course, you could just use a number.

Date: The date that you added the SCOBY to this particular batch.

Fermentation Vessel: If you are using more than one fermenter at a time, you will need to designate which one this batch of kombucha is being brewed in. You can use a name, number, a description, or just the volume of the vessel.

Location: Kombucha does best when allowed to brew undisturbed, away from other fermenting foods, cooking areas, sunlight and contaminants. As you try out different locations some will prove to be better places than others to set your brew, so write it down.

Observations chart: As each batch of kombucha progresses, you will want to make some notes about them. Temperature has a major effect on how long your brew takes to mature, as well as the final taste. It is a good idea to take daily temperature readings, but you can do as many as you want and write them in here. You might also record the pH of the solution. The *Observations chart* is where you would also record changes that you notice in your SCOBY.

Recipe Index

Write the name of the flavor you created and the page it is located on and, after you have enjoyed your kombucha, you can also rate it on this page. By doing so, you will easily know which recipes were your favorites.

Fermentation 2 Recipe Pages

This is the place to record the flavorings for fermentation 2 whether in bottles or a secondary fermentation vessel. Write down what fruits, herbs, or other additions were added, how much, and how they were prepared. Did you grate ginger or slice it? Pulverize fruits in a blender or chop them? Use fresh or dried herbs?

Also, record the things you notice about the appearance in the bottles. How does the color look? How much head space did you leave?

Then note how many days until ready for drinking and all of your notes about fizz, flavor and what you might change next time.

If you love this flavor, be sure and note that in the recipe index in the front using your own rating system.

Recipe Pages Fields (see completed sample form on page 11)

Getting Started

Recipe Name: Enter the name of your recipe here. You can use a descriptive name, like Blueberry Ginger, or create a fun, unique name, such as Bambucha.

Date: This is where you write in the date that you are starting your secondary fermentation by adding fruit, herbs, etc. to your finished kombucha to flavor it.

From Batch/Page #: Each recipe is created from a specific batch. In this space put down which batch you are creating this recipe from. You can write in the batch number, page number or both.

From SCOBY : Record which SCOBY created the batch of kombucha used in this recipe.

Ingredient Table

Date : You will usually add all the flavoring ingredients at the same time, so the date fields will all be the same as the date at the top of this page. If you do decide to add an ingredient later, you can write in the date in these spaces.

Ingredient: Record the name of each of the ingredients you are using to flavor your kombucha. Be as descriptive as possible so that you can make changes or recreate the recipe next time, exactly. For example, you might write, "Fresh organic strawberries from Meyer's farm stand, chopped."

Amount: The amount of each ingredient goes in this space. You might also want to indicate the size of the container that the ingredient is flavoring, such as ¼ cup/16 oz.

Daily Observations: It is useful to check on your recipe every day or two to see if it is ready to refrigerate and enjoy. You can record your observations in these spaces. For each observation you may want to put down the date and perhaps the time.

Bottling Table

Number: Write down the number of bottles you created with this recipe.

Volume: Are you using 16 oz. bottles, 1 Liter bottles or another size? Write that in this space so you know your total kombucha yield for this recipe.

Type: There are many types of bottles which can be used for a secondary fermentation of kombucha. You can record that information here. For instance, you may be using plastic, 1 Liter soda bottles. If so, write that here so you will remember.

Tasting Notes

Each batch of kombucha is unique and each recipe of flavoring agents produces a unique product. This is where you will write down how this recipe tasted to you. Was it fizzy enough, too sweet, too sour or just perfect? Record you tasting notes here so that you can recreate your best recipes again and again.

SCOBY Family Tree Pages

The SCOBY that you start with is called the Mother. Each time you brew, the Mother will grow a new baby on top. After a few batches you will want to separate the new babies from the mother. So, before you know it you will have two -then increasingly more SCOBYs. You will want to keep track of them so that you can decide which ones to retire or compost or just save in a SCOBY Hotel for future brewing.

If you experiment with ingredients like coffee, essential oils, or other flavorings that change or damage the SCOBY you will want to record that and keep that SCOBY out of future brews. Use the Kombucha Flow Chart model to help you (see chart on page 102).

SCOBY Name: is where you create a designation for your SCOBY. Some SCOBYs come with a known lineage name, but feel free to name it anything you want, or just give it a number.

SCOBY Mother: If this SCOBY is the baby of another one, write in the SCOBY from which it grew here to keep track of the lineage of your SCOBYs.

Acquired Date and Source: Enter the date you received your SCOBY and where you got it.

The next part of the form is for you to record each time you create a batch of kombucha with this SCOBY by entering the date you began the brew, which page of the brew record it was used for, the type of brew (tea, coffee, or specialty).

Date: Write in the date that you started each batch of kombucha with this SCOBY.

Brewing Record Page #: Record the brewing record page number for each batch of kombucha that you made with this SCOBY

Type of Brew: This space is for you to write in what type of kombucha that you made with this SCOBY. It will most often be sweet tea, but you there are other specialized ingredients that you can use to brew kombucha. If you use them, write them here so that you know the kind of kombucha this SCOBY was used to brew.

Notes: This space is for any additional information or observations that you want to remember for this SCOBY. You can make notes about appearance, if it is was placed on hold in a hotel for a while and so forth.

Inspirations Pages

Keep track of random ideas here. Got an idea for a future recipe? This is a great place to jot that down. Did you learn something new on a forum? Note it here. Use this as a place to capture anything kombucha related, including stories about places you tasted kombucha, sharing kombucha with newbies, giving your child their first sips, and more.

Getting Started

Wellness Diary Pages

Most people who drink kombucha are interested in their health and wellness. Make a note of the date you started brewing (or journaling) and your personal wellness goals. If you are sharing this journal just leave room for the whole household to record their starting date and goals. Then come back to these pages to write about positive changes as you notice them.

Goals some folks have are as simple as cutting back on soda or sugar. Others are looking for improved digestion, better skin texture, healing joint pain and more. Your wellness goals are up to you, but it helps to keep track of successes as we often forget our challenges once they are gone.

Use this section to help you to know how much kombucha to drink, as well. Find the best times of day and amounts for your body.

Purchase Record Pages

Keep track of the sources for ingredients, price paid and your satisfaction level for the item here. You may want to reorder that favorite tea and want good records for where it came from. You may want to figure out just how much your home brewed kombucha costs you and how often you want to purchase tea, sugar or other ingredients.

Kombucha Brewing Flow Chart

On the following page is a diagram to help explain the kombucha brewing process and the need for careful records. As you will see, each batch of kombucha is made with particular ingredients, brewed in a certain manner and fermented by a specific SCOBY.

The completed batch of kombucha can then be made into any number of recipes with a secondary fermentation that can include any number of flavoring ingredients. This journal will help you keep track of each batch of kombucha that you brew, each recipe that you create and each SCOBY that is formed during the fermentation process.

We love the process of brewing kombucha and enjoy drinking it on a daily basis. It is our hope that you will come to enjoy it as much as we do. Have fun!

Neil & Laurie Stolmaker

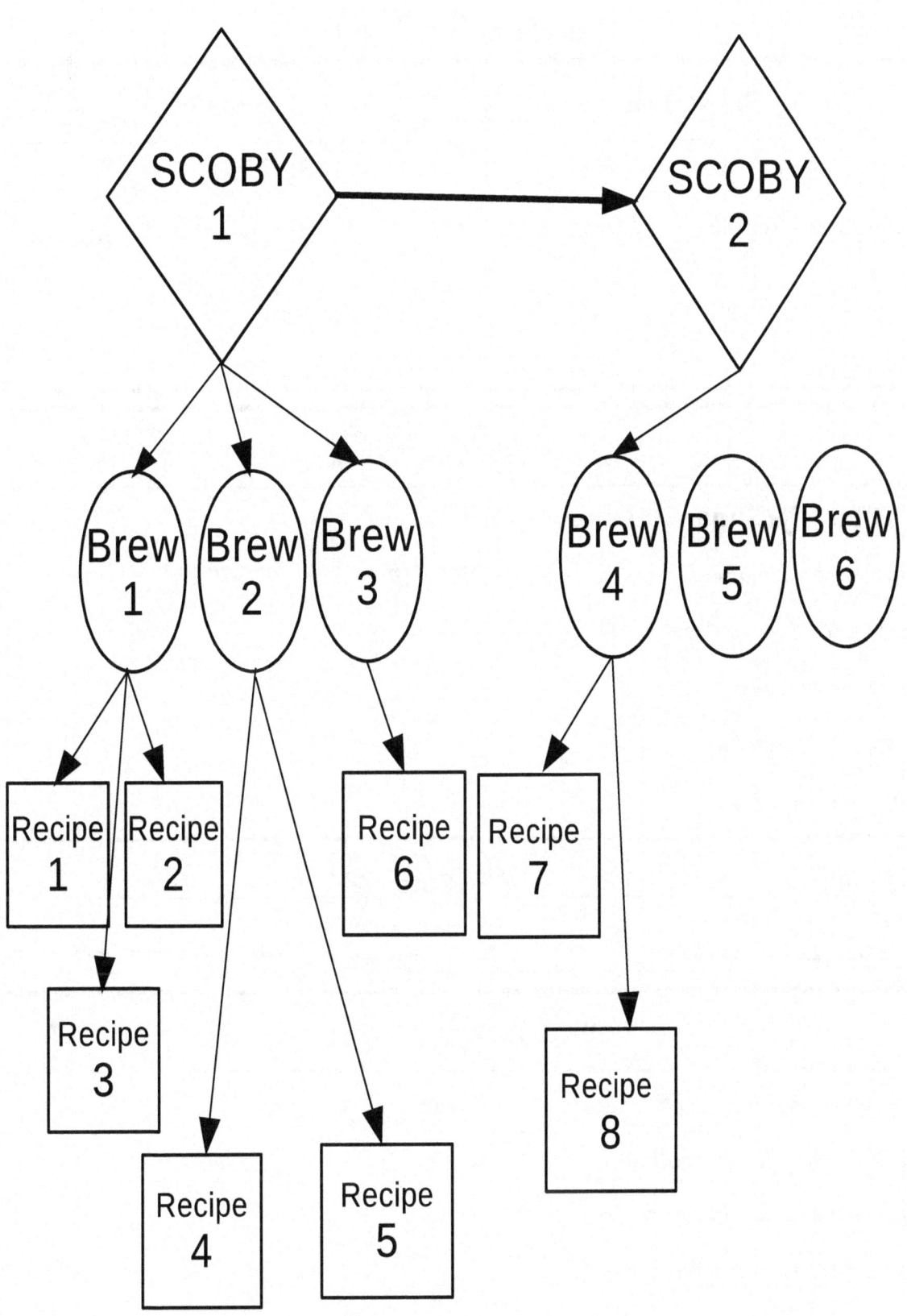

Brewing Records

Batch# __5__ (BB)/ CB   Previous Batch#/Page# __3__

Date Begun: __02/12/16__   Date Bottled: __02/21/16__

Ingredient	Amount	Brew Time
Yunnan Fannings Black Tea	3 Tblsp	10 min
Chinese Green Fannings Tea	2 Tblsp	10 min
Organic white sugar	1 cup	

Steps

Added: ☒ Tea ☒ Sugar ☐ Other:

Boiled 8 cups filtered water	wrapped heat mat around jar
Brewed tea for 10 min	
Added 1 cup organic sugar	
Cooled to room temperature	
added to 2 Gal fermenter	

SCOBY name: __Alpha 1__   Date: __02/12/16__

Fermentation vessel: __2 Gal glass__   Location: __kitchen counter corner__

Observations

Temperature after 24 hours 78°
02/14 SCOBY looking a bit thicker
02/16 small bubbles seen in fermenter
02/19 tastes sour, seems almost ready
02/21 Bottled 14 x 16oz bottles

Recipes

Recipe Name: Blueberry Ginger **Date:** 02/21/16

From Batch/Page# 5 **From SCOBY:** apha 1

Date	Ingredient	Amount
02/21	frozen blueberries, thawed	2 Tblsp
"	whole ginger root, sliced in 1" rounds	2

Daily Observations

02/23 not much fizz yet	
02/25 getting fizzy, burped bottles	
02/28 plenty fizzy	
02/28 refregerated all bottles	

Bottles

Number	Volume	Type
14	16 oz	GT's with new lids

Tasting Notes

some ginger punch, some blueberry flavor, Nice fizz
03/02 flavor has mellowed. More blueberry flavor, mellow ginger
next time: try chopping blueberries and adding more ginger

http://kombuchajournal.com   11

Brewing Records

Batch# _____   BB   CB   Previous Batch#/Page# _____

Date Begun: _____   Date Bottled: _____

Ingredient	Amount	Brew Time

Steps
Added: ☐ Tea   ☐ Sugar   ☐ Other: _____

SCOBY name: _____   Date: _____

Fermentation vessel: _____   Location: _____

Observations

Brewing Records

Batch# _____   BB   CB   Previous Batch#/Page# _____

Date Begun: _____   Date Bottled: _____

Ingredient	Amount	Brew Time

Steps
Added: ☐ **Tea**   ☐ **Sugar**   ☐ **Other**:

SCOBY name: _____   Date: _____

Fermentation vessel: _____   Location: _____

Observations

Brewing Records

Batch# _____   BB   CB   Previous Batch#/Page# _____

Date Begun: _____   Date Bottled: _____

Ingredient	Amount	Brew Time

Steps
Added: ☐ **Tea**   ☐ **Sugar**   ☐ **Other**:

SCOBY name: _____   Date: _____

Fermentation vessel: _____   Location: _____

Observations

Brewing Records

Batch# _____   BB CB   Previous Batch#/Page# _____

Date Begun: _____   Date Bottled: _____

Ingredient	Amount	Brew Time

Steps

Added: ☐ Tea   ☐ Sugar   ☐ Other: _____

SCOBY name: _____   Date: _____

Fermentation vessel: _____   Location: _____

Observations

http://kombuchajournal.com

Brewing Records

Batch# _____   BB   CB   Previous Batch#/Page# _____

Date Begun: _____   Date Bottled: _____

Ingredient	Amount	Brew Time

Steps
Added: ☐ **Tea**   ☐ **Sugar**   ☐ **Other**:

SCOBY name: _____   Date: _____

Fermentation vessel: _____   Location: _____

Observations

Brewing Records

Batch# _____   BB   CB   Previous Batch#/Page# _____

Date Begun: _____   Date Bottled: _____

Ingredient	Amount	Brew Time

Steps
Added: ☐ **Tea**   ☐ **Sugar**   ☐ **Other**:

SCOBY name: _____   Date: _____

Fermentation vessel: _____   Location: _____

Observations

http://kombuchajournal.com

Brewing Records

Batch# _____   BB   CB   Previous Batch#/Page# _____

Date Begun: _____   Date Bottled: _____

Ingredient	Amount	Brew Time

Steps

Added: ☐ **Tea**   ☐ **Sugar**   ☐ **Other**: _____

SCOBY name: _____   Date: _____

Fermentation vessel: _____   Location: _____

Observations

Brewing Records

Batch# _____   BB   CB   Previous Batch#/Page# _____

Date Begun: _____   Date Bottled: _____

Ingredient	Amount	Brew Time

Steps
Added: ☐ Tea   ☐ Sugar   ☐ Other:

SCOBY name: _____   Date: _____

Fermentation vessel: _____   Location: _____

Observations

http://kombuchajournal.com

Brewing Records

Batch# _____   BB   CB   Previous Batch#/Page# _____

Date Begun: _____   Date Bottled: _____

Ingredient	Amount	Brew Time

Steps

Added: ☐ **Tea**   ☐ **Sugar**   ☐ **Other**:

SCOBY name: _____   Date: _____

Fermentation vessel: _____   Location: _____

Observations

Brewing Records

Batch# _____   BB   CB   Previous Batch#/Page# _____

Date Begun: _____   Date Bottled: _____

Ingredient	Amount	Brew Time

Steps
Added: ☐ **Tea**   ☐ **Sugar**   ☐ **Other**:

SCOBY name: _____   Date: _____

Fermentation vessel: _____   Location: _____

Observations

http://kombuchajournal.com

Brewing Records

Batch# _____   BB   CB   Previous Batch#/Page# _____

Date Begun: _____   Date Bottled: _____

Ingredient	Amount	Brew Time

Steps
Added: ☐ **Tea**   ☐ **Sugar**   ☐ **Other**:

SCOBY name: _____   Date: _____

Fermentation vessel: _____   Location: _____

Observations

Brewing Records

Batch# _____   BB   CB   Previous Batch#/Page# _____

Date Begun: _____   Date Bottled: _____

Ingredient	Amount	Brew Time

Steps
Added: ☐ Tea   ☐ Sugar   ☐ Other: _____

SCOBY name: _____   Date: _____

Fermentation vessel: _____   Location: _____

Observations

Brewing Records

Batch# _____   BB   CB   Previous Batch#/Page# _____

Date Begun: _____   Date Bottled: _____

Ingredient	Amount	Brew Time

Steps

Added: ☐ Tea   ☐ Sugar   ☐ Other: _____

SCOBY name: _____   Date: _____

Fermentation vessel: _____   Location: _____

Observations

Brewing Records

Batch# _____   BB   CB   Previous Batch#/Page# _____

Date Begun: _____   Date Bottled: _____

Ingredient	Amount	Brew Time

Steps

Added: ☐ **Tea**   ☐ **Sugar**   ☐ **Other**: _____

SCOBY name: _____   Date: _____

Fermentation vessel: _____   Location: _____

Observations

http://kombuchajournal.com

Brewing Records

Batch# _____   BB   CB   Previous Batch#/Page# _____

Date Begun: _____   Date Bottled: _____

Ingredient	Amount	Brew Time

Steps

Added: ☐ Tea   ☐ Sugar   ☐ Other:

SCOBY name: _____   Date: _____

Fermentation vessel: _____   Location: _____

Observations

Brewing Records

Batch# _____   BB   CB   Previous Batch#/Page# _____

Date Begun: _____   Date Bottled: _____

Ingredient	Amount	Brew Time

Steps
Added: ☐ **Tea**   ☐ **Sugar**   ☐ **Other**:

SCOBY name: _____   Date: _____

Fermentation vessel: _____   Location: _____

Observations

Brewing Records

Batch# _____   BB   CB   Previous Batch#/Page# _____

Date Begun: _____   Date Bottled: _____

Ingredient	Amount	Brew Time

Steps
Added: ☐ Tea   ☐ Sugar   ☐ Other: _____

SCOBY name: _____   Date: _____

Fermentation vessel: _____   Location: _____

Observations

http://kombuchajournal.com

Brewing Records

Batch# _____   BB   CB   Previous Batch#/Page# _____

Date Begun: _____   Date Bottled: _____

Ingredient	Amount	Brew Time

Steps

Added: ☐ **Tea**   ☐ **Sugar**   ☐ **Other**: _____

SCOBY name: _____   Date: _____

Fermentation vessel: _____   Location: _____

Observations

Brewing Records

Batch# _____   BB   CB   Previous Batch#/Page# _____

Date Begun: _____   Date Bottled: _____

Ingredient	Amount	Brew Time

Steps
Added: ☐ Tea   ☐ Sugar   ☐ Other:

SCOBY name: _____   Date: _____

Fermentation vessel: _____   Location: _____

Observations

Brewing Records

Batch# _____   BB   CB   Previous Batch#/Page# _____

Date Begun: _____   Date Bottled: _____

Ingredient	Amount	Brew Time

Steps
Added: ☐ Tea   ☐ Sugar   ☐ Other:

SCOBY name: _____   Date: _____

Fermentation vessel: _____   Location: _____

Observations

http://kombuchajournal.com

Brewing Records

Batch# _____   BB   CB   Previous Batch#/Page# _____

Date Begun: _____   Date Bottled: _____

Ingredient	Amount	Brew Time

Steps

Added: ☐ Tea   ☐ Sugar   ☐ Other: _____

SCOBY name: _____   Date: _____

Fermentation vessel: _____   Location: _____

Observations

Brewing Records

Batch# _____   BB   CB   Previous Batch#/Page# _____

Date Begun: _____   Date Bottled: _____

Ingredient	Amount	Brew Time

Steps

Added: ☐ **Tea**   ☐ **Sugar**   ☐ **Other**: _____

SCOBY name: _____   Date: _____

Fermentation vessel: _____   Location: _____

Observations

Brewing Records

Batch# _____   BB   CB   Previous Batch#/Page# _____

Date Begun: _____   Date Bottled: _____

Ingredient	Amount	Brew Time

Steps

Added: ☐ **Tea**   ☐ **Sugar**   ☐ **Other:**

SCOBY name: _____   Date: _____

Fermentation vessel: _____   Location: _____

Observations

Brewing Records

Batch# _____   BB   CB   Previous Batch#/Page# _____

Date Begun: _____   Date Bottled: _____

Ingredient	Amount	Brew Time

Steps

Added: ☐ Tea   ☐ Sugar   ☐ Other: _____

SCOBY name: _____   Date: _____

Fermentation vessel: _____   Location: _____

Observations

http://kombuchajournal.com

Brewing Records

Batch# _____   BB   CB   Previous Batch#/Page# _____

Date Begun: _____   Date Bottled: _____

Ingredient	Amount	Brew Time

Steps
Added: ☐ **Tea**   ☐ **Sugar**   ☐ **Other**:

SCOBY name: _____   Date: _____

Fermentation vessel: _____   Location: _____

Observations

Brewing Records

Batch# _____   BB   CB   Previous Batch#/Page# _____

Date Begun: _____   Date Bottled: _____

Ingredient	Amount	Brew Time

Steps
Added: ☐ **Tea**   ☐ **Sugar**   ☐ **Other:**

SCOBY name: _____   Date: _____

Fermentation vessel: _____   Location: _____

Observations

Brewing Records

Batch# _____   BB   CB   Previous Batch#/Page# _____

Date Begun: _____   Date Bottled: _____

Ingredient	Amount	Brew Time

Steps
Added: ☐ Tea   ☐ Sugar   ☐ Other:

SCOBY name: _____   Date: _____

Fermentation vessel: _____   Location: _____

Observations

38   http://kombuchajournal.com

Brewing Records

Batch#_____   BB   CB   Previous Batch#/Page# _____

Date Begun: _____   Date Bottled: _____

Ingredient	Amount	Brew Time

Steps
Added: ☐ **Tea**   ☐ **Sugar**   ☐ **Other**:

SCOBY name: _____   Date: _____

Fermentation vessel: _____   Location: _____

Observations

http://kombuchajournal.com

Brewing Records

Batch# _____   BB   CB   Previous Batch#/Page# _____

Date Begun: _____   Date Bottled: _____

Ingredient	Amount	Brew Time

Steps

Added: ☐ Tea   ☐ Sugar   ☐ Other: _____

SCOBY name: _____   Date: _____

Fermentation vessel: _____   Location: _____

Observations

Brewing Records

Batch# _____ BB CB Previous Batch#/Page# _____

Date Begun: _____ Date Bottled: _____

Ingredient	Amount	Brew Time

Steps

Added: ☐ **Tea**   ☐ **Sugar**   ☐ **Other**: _____

SCOBY name: _____ Date: _____

Fermentation vessel: _____ Location: _____

Observations

Brewing Records

Batch# _____   BB   CB   Previous Batch#/Page# _____

Date Begun: _____   Date Bottled: _____

Ingredient	Amount	Brew Time

Steps
Added: ☐ **Tea**   ☐ **Sugar**   ☐ **Other**:

SCOBY name: _____   Date: _____

Fermentation vessel: _____   Location: _____

Observations

Brewing Records

Batch#_____   BB   CB   Previous Batch#/Page# _____

Date Begun: _____   Date Bottled: _____

Ingredient	Amount	Brew Time

Steps

Added: ☐ Tea   ☐ Sugar   ☐ Other: _____

SCOBY name: _____   Date: _____

Fermentation vessel: _____   Location: _____

Observations

http://kombuchajournal.com   43

Brewing Records

Batch# _____   BB   CB   Previous Batch#/Page# _____

Date Begun: _____   Date Bottled: _____

Ingredient	Amount	Brew Time

Steps
Added: ☐ Tea   ☐ Sugar   ☐ Other:

SCOBY name: _____   Date: _____

Fermentation vessel: _____   Location: _____

Observations

44   http://kombuchajournal.com

Brewing Records

Batch# _____   BB   CB   Previous Batch#/Page# _____

Date Begun: _____   Date Bottled: _____

Ingredient	Amount	Brew Time

Steps
Added: ☐ **Tea**   ☐ **Sugar**   ☐ **Other**:

SCOBY name: _____   Date: _____

Fermentation vessel: _____   Location: _____

Observations

http://kombuchajournal.com

Brewing Records

Batch# _____   BB   CB   Previous Batch#/Page# _____

Date Begun: _____   Date Bottled: _____

Ingredient	Amount	Brew Time

Steps
Added: ☐ **Tea**   ☐ **Sugar**   ☐ **Other**:

SCOBY name: _____   Date: _____

Fermentation vessel: _____   Location: _____

Observations

Brewing Records

Batch# _____   BB   CB   Previous Batch#/Page# _____

Date Begun: _____   Date Bottled: _____

Ingredient	Amount	Brew Time

Steps
Added: ☐ **Tea**   ☐ **Sugar**   ☐ **Other**:

SCOBY name: _____   Date: _____

Fermentation vessel: _____   Location: _____

Observations

http://kombuchajournal.com

Brewing Records

Batch# _____   BB   CB   Previous Batch#/Page# _____

Date Begun: _____   Date Bottled: _____

Ingredient	Amount	Brew Time

Steps
Added: ☐ **Tea**   ☐ **Sugar**   ☐ **Other:**

SCOBY name: _____   Date: _____

Fermentation vessel: _____   Location: _____

Observations

48   http://kombuchajournal.com

Brewing Records

Batch# _____   BB   CB   Previous Batch#/Page# _____

Date Begun: _____   Date Bottled: _____

Ingredient	Amount	Brew Time

Steps

Added: ☐ **Tea**   ☐ **Sugar**   ☐ **Other:**

SCOBY name: _____   Date: _____

Fermentation vessel: _____   Location: _____

Observations

http://kombuchajournal.com   49

Brewing Records

Batch# _____   BB   CB   Previous Batch#/Page# _____

Date Begun: _____   Date Bottled: _____

Ingredient	Amount	Brew Time

Steps
Added: ☐ **Tea**   ☐ **Sugar**   ☐ **Other**:

SCOBY name: _____   Date: _____

Fermentation vessel: _____   Location: _____

Observations

50   http://kombuchajournal.com

Brewing Records

Batch# _____   BB   CB   Previous Batch#/Page# _____

Date Begun: _____   Date Bottled: _____

Ingredient	Amount	Brew Time

Steps
Added: ☐ **Tea**   ☐ **Sugar**   ☐ **Other**:

SCOBY name: _____   Date: _____

Fermentation vessel: _____   Location: _____

Observations

Brewing Records

Batch# _____   BB   CB   Previous Batch#/Page# _____

Date Begun: _____   Date Bottled: _____

Ingredient	Amount	Brew Time

Steps
Added: ☐ **Tea**   ☐ **Sugar**   ☐ **Other**:

SCOBY name: _____   Date: _____

Fermentation vessel: _____   Location: _____

Observations

Brewing Records

Batch# _____   BB   CB   Previous Batch#/Page# _____

Date Begun: _____   Date Bottled: _____

Ingredient	Amount	Brew Time

Steps

Added: ☐ **Tea**   ☐ **Sugar**   ☐ **Other**: _____

SCOBY name: _____   Date: _____

Fermentation vessel: _____   Location: _____

Observations

http://kombuchajournal.com

Brewing Records

Batch# _____   BB   CB   Previous Batch#/Page# _____

Date Begun: _____   Date Bottled: _____

Ingredient	Amount	Brew Time

Steps
Added: ☐ **Tea**   ☐ **Sugar**   ☐ **Other**:

SCOBY name: _____   Date: _____

Fermentation vessel: _____   Location: _____

Observations

http://kombuchajournal.com

Brewing Records

Batch# _____   BB   CB   Previous Batch#/Page# _____

Date Begun: _____   Date Bottled: _____

Ingredient	Amount	Brew Time

Steps
Added: ☐ Tea   ☐ Sugar   ☐ Other:

SCOBY name: _____   Date: _____

Fermentation vessel: _____   Location: _____

Observations

http://kombuchajournal.com

Brewing Records

Batch# _____   BB   CB   Previous Batch#/Page# _____

Date Begun: _____   Date Bottled: _____

Ingredient	Amount	Brew Time

Steps
Added: ☐ **Tea**   ☐ **Sugar**   ☐ **Other**:

SCOBY name: _____   Date: _____

Fermentation vessel: _____   Location: _____

Observations

Brewing Records

Batch# _____   BB   CB   Previous Batch#/Page# _____

Date Begun: _____   Date Bottled: _____

Ingredient	Amount	Brew Time

Steps

Added: ☐ **Tea**   ☐ **Sugar**   ☐ **Other**: _____

SCOBY name: _____   Date: _____

Fermentation vessel: _____   Location: _____

Observations

http://kombuchajournal.com

Brewing Records

Batch# _____   BB   CB   Previous Batch#/Page# _____

Date Begun: _____   Date Bottled: _____

Ingredient	Amount	Brew Time

Steps
Added: ☐ **Tea**   ☐ **Sugar**   ☐ **Other**:

SCOBY name: _____   Date: _____

Fermentation vessel: _____   Location: _____

Observations

Brewing Records

Batch# _____ BB CB Previous Batch#/Page# _____

Date Begun: _____ Date Bottled: _____

Ingredient	Amount	Brew Time

Steps

Added: ☐ **Tea** ☐ **Sugar** ☐ **Other**: _____

SCOBY name: _____ Date: _____

Fermentation vessel: _____ Location: _____

Observations

Recipes

Date	Recipe Name	Page number	Rating

Recipes

Date	Recipe Name	Page number	Rating

Recipes

Recipe Name: _____ Date: _____

From Batch/Page#: _____ From SCOBY _____

Date	Ingredient	Amount

Daily Observations

Bottles		
Number	Volume	Type

Tasting Notes

Recipes

Recipe Name: _____   Date: _____

From Batch/Page#: _____   From SCOBY _____

Date	Ingredient	Amount

Daily Observations

Bottles		
Number	**Volume**	**Type**

Tasting Notes

Recipes

Recipe Name: _____   Date: _____

From Batch/Page# _____   From SCOBY: _____

Date	Ingredient	Amount

Daily Observations

Bottles		
Number	Volume	Type

Tasting Notes

Recipes

Recipe Name: _____   Date: _____

From Batch/Page# _____   From SCOBY: _____

Date	Ingredient	Amount

Daily Observations

Bottles		
Number	Volume	Type

Tasting Notes

Recipes

Recipe Name: _____ Date: _____

From Batch/Page# _____ From SCOBY: _____

Date	Ingredient	Amount

Daily Observations

Bottles

Number	Volume	Type

Tasting Notes

Recipes

Recipe Name: _____ Date:_____

From Batch/Page# _____ From SCOBY: _____

Date	Ingredient	Amount

Daily Observations

Bottles

Number	Volume	Type

Tasting Notes

Recipes

Recipe Name: _____   Date: _____

From Batch/Page# _____   From SCOBY: _____

Date	Ingredient	Amount

Daily Observations

Bottles

Number	Volume	Type

Tasting Notes

Recipes

Recipe Name: _____ Date: _____

From Batch/Page# _____ From SCOBY: _____

Date	Ingredient	Amount

Daily Observations

Bottles		
Number	**Volume**	**Type**

Tasting Notes

Recipes

Recipe Name: _____ Date: _____

From Batch/Page# _____ From SCOBY: _____

Date	Ingredient	Amount

Daily Observations

Bottles		
Number	Volume	Type

Tasting Notes

Recipes

Recipe Name: _____   Date: _____

From Batch/Page# _____   From SCOBY: _____

Date	Ingredient	Amount

Daily Observations

Bottles		
Number	**Volume**	**Type**

Tasting Notes

http://kombuchajournal.com

Recipes

Recipe Name: _____   Date: _____

From Batch/Page# _____   From SCOBY: _____

Date	Ingredient	Amount

Daily Observations

Bottles		
Number	Volume	Type

Tasting Notes

Recipes

Recipe Name: _____   Date: _____

From Batch/Page# _____   From SCOBY: _____

Date	Ingredient	Amount

Daily Observations

Bottles		
Number	Volume	Type

Tasting Notes

Recipes

Recipe Name: _____ Date: _____

From Batch/Page# _____ From SCOBY: _____

Date	Ingredient	Amount

Daily Observations

Bottles		
Number	Volume	Type

Tasting Notes

Recipes

Recipe Name: _____   Date:_____

From Batch/Page# _____   From SCOBY: _____

Date	Ingredient	Amount

Daily Observations

Bottles		
Number	**Volume**	**Type**

Tasting Notes

http://kombuchajournal.com

Recipes

Recipe Name: _____ Date: _____

From Batch/Page# _____ From SCOBY: _____

Date	Ingredient	Amount

Daily Observations

Bottles		
Number	Volume	Type

Tasting Notes

Recipes

Recipe Name: _____   Date: _____

From Batch/Page# _____   From SCOBY: _____

Date	Ingredient	Amount

Daily Observations

Bottles		
Number	Volume	Type

Tasting Notes

Recipes

Recipe Name: _____ Date: _____

From Batch/Page# _____ From SCOBY: _____

Date	Ingredient	Amount

Daily Observations

Bottles

Number	Volume	Type

Tasting Notes

http://kombuchajournal.com

Recipes

Recipe Name: _____   Date: _____

From Batch/Page# _____   From SCOBY: _____

Date	Ingredient	Amount

Daily Observations

Bottles		
Number	**Volume**	**Type**

Tasting Notes

Recipes

Recipe Name: _____ Date: _____

From Batch/Page# _____ From SCOBY: _____

Date	Ingredient	Amount

Daily Observations

Bottles		
Number	Volume	Type

Tasting Notes

Recipes

Recipe Name: _____   Date: _____

From Batch/Page# _____   From SCOBY: _____

Date	Ingredient	Amount

Daily Observations

Bottles		
Number	Volume	Type

Tasting Notes

http://kombuchajournal.com

Recipes

Recipe Name: _____   Date: _____

From Batch/Page# _____   From SCOBY: _____

Date	Ingredient	Amount

Daily Observations

Bottles		
Number	Volume	Type

Tasting Notes

Recipes

Recipe Name: _____ Date: _____

From Batch/Page# _____ From SCOBY: _____

Date	Ingredient	Amount

Daily Observations

Bottles		
Number	Volume	Type

Tasting Notes

Recipes

Recipe Name: _____   Date: _____

From Batch/Page# _____   From SCOBY: _____

Date	Ingredient	Amount

Daily Observations

Bottles		
Number	Volume	Type

Tasting Notes

Recipes

Recipe Name: _____   Date: _____

From Batch/Page# _____   From SCOBY: _____

Date	Ingredient	Amount

Daily Observations

Bottles

Number	Volume	Type

Tasting Notes

SCOBY Family Tree

SCOBY Name: _____   SCOBY Mother: _____

Aquired Date/Source: _____

Date	Brewing Record Page#	Type of Brew

Notes

SCOBY Family Tree

SCOBY Name: _____   SCOBY Mother: _____

Aquired Date/Source: _____

Date	Brewing Record Page#	Type of Brew

Notes

SCOBY Family Tree

SCOBY Name: _____   SCOBY Mother: _____

Aquired Date/Source: _____

Date	Brewing Record Page#	Type of Brew

Notes

SCOBY Family Tree

SCOBY Name: _____   SCOBY Mother: _____

Aquired Date/Source: _____

Date	Brewing Record Page#	Type of Brew

Notes

SCOBY Family Tree

SCOBY Name: _____   SCOBY Mother: _____

Aquired Date/Source: _____

Date	Brewing Record Page#	Type of Brew

Notes

SCOBY Family Tree

SCOBY Name: _____ SCOBY Mother: _____

Aquired Date/Source: _____

Date	Brewing Record Page#	Type of Brew

Notes

SCOBY Family Tree

SCOBY Name: _____   SCOBY Mother: _____

Aquired Date/Source: _____

Date	Brewing Record Page#	Type of Brew

Notes

SCOBY Family Tree

SCOBY Name: _____   SCOBY Mother: _____

Aquired Date/Source: _____

Date	Brewing Record Page#	Type of Brew

Notes

SCOBY Family Tree

SCOBY Name: _____   SCOBY Mother: _____

Aquired Date/Source: _____

Date	Brewing Record Page#	Type of Brew

Notes

SCOBY Family Tree

SCOBY Name: _____   SCOBY Mother: _____

Aquired Date/Source:_____

Date	Brewing Record Page#	Type of Brew

Notes

Inspirations

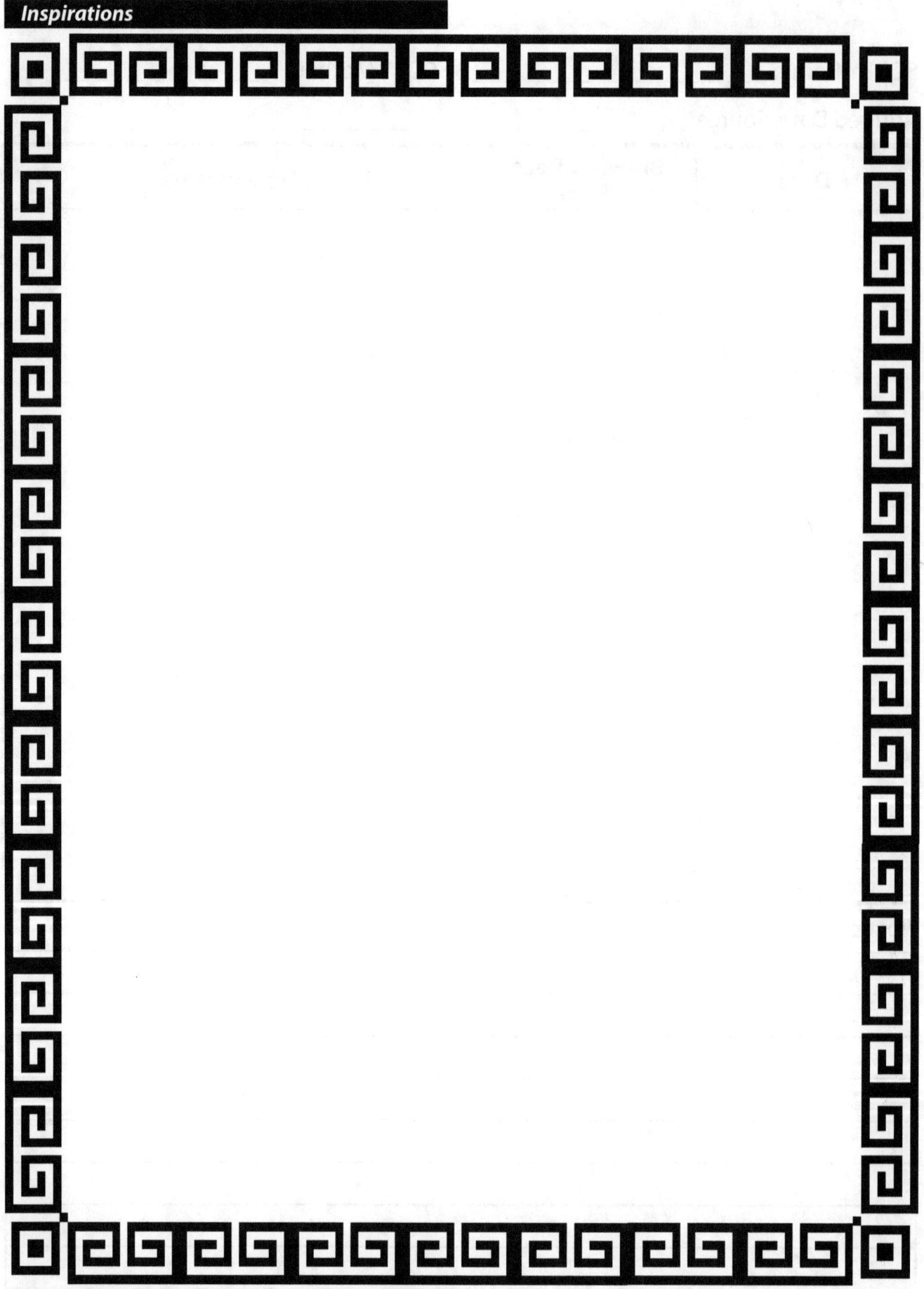

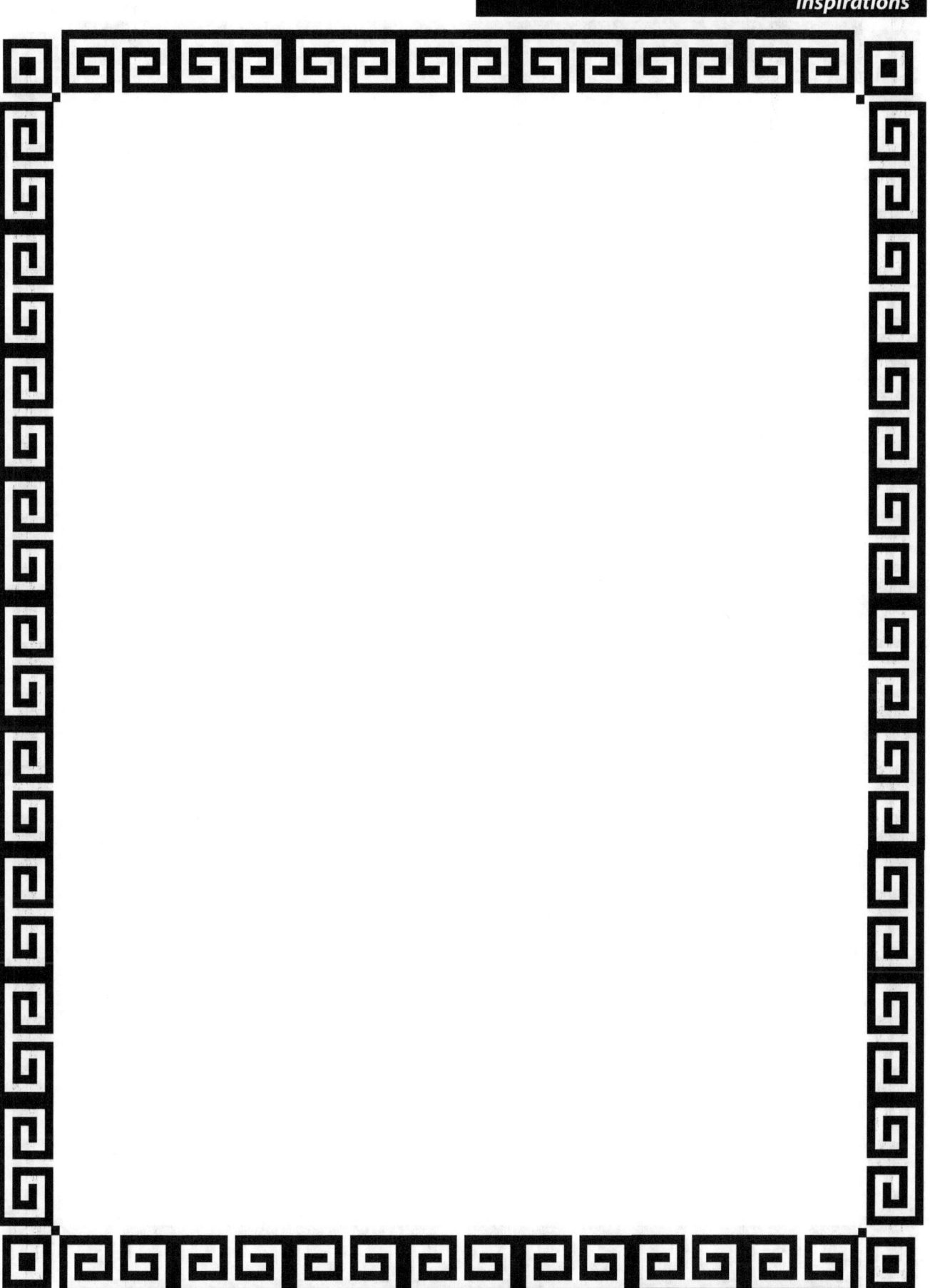

Inspirations

Inspirations

http://kombuchajournal.com

Wellness Notes

Wellness Notes

Wellness Notes

Wellness Notes

Purchases

Date	Item	Source	Cost

Purchases

Date	Item	Source	Cost

www.ingramcontent.com/pod-product-compliance
Lightning Source LLC
Chambersburg PA
CBHW060517300426
44112CB00017B/2705